THE SILENT INVADERS

A Comprehensive Guide to Eliminating
Parasites for Optimal Health

RENE MULBERY

ISBN: 9798387088766

Cover design by: Rene Mulbery
Library of Congress Control Number: 2018675309
Printed in the United States of America

CONTENTS

Title Page

Copyright

Dedication

Introduction

Chapter 1: Understanding Parasites   1

Chapter 2: Natural Remedies for Eliminating Parasites   10

Chapter 3: Medical Treatments for Parasite Infections   25

Chapter 4: Detoxification and Cleansing   35

Chapter 5: Restoring Health After Parasite Infections   43

Chapter 6: Prevention and Maintenance   53

Conclusion   60

Final thoughts   64

Acknowledgment   67

DEDICATION

To all those who are striving to maintain a healthy lifestyle in a world filled with processed and unhealthy food, I dedicate my utmost admiration and respect. The journey to good health is not an uncomplicated one, but your dedication and commitment to prioritizing your well-being are truly inspiring.

In a world where fast food and convenience products are the norm, it takes heroic effort and discipline to choose healthy and wholesome foods. Your determination to make these choices and prioritize your health is a testament to your strength and resilience.

I commend your efforts to use resources that support your health, such as nutrition education, exercise programs, and wellness practices. Your willingness to learn and grow in these areas is a testament to your dedication to living a healthy and fulfilling life.

As someone who understands the challenges of maintaining a healthy lifestyle, I offer my support and encouragement to you on your journey. May you continue to make positive choices for your

health and inspire others to do the same.
Thank you for your dedication to staying healthy in a world that often makes it difficult. Your efforts are deeply appreciated and valued.

INTRODUCTION

Parasites are organisms that live on or inside a host organism and derive their nutrition from it. They can range in size from microscopic single-celled organisms to large multi-cellular organisms visible to the naked eye. They found parasites in every corner of the globe, and they can infect humans, animals, and plants.

Parasites can harm the body in several ways. Some parasites can cause damage by physically attaching to or invading host tissues, while others can cause harm by producing toxins or by interfering with normal body functions. Parasites can cause a wide range of health problems, including digestive disorders, anemia, malnutrition, and even death.

The history of parasites is long and complex. Parasites have been present throughout the history of life on Earth, and they have evolved alongside their hosts over millions of years. Some researchers believe that parasites have played a key role in shaping the evolution of their hosts.

There are various examples of parasites that have had a significant impact on human history. One of the most famous examples is the Plasmodium parasite, which causes malaria. Malaria has been a major public health problem for centuries, and it continues to be a major cause of illness and death in many parts of the world. Another example is tapeworms, which can cause they can transmit considerable damage to the digestive system and humans through contaminated food.

Despite the significant harm that parasites can cause, they are also important components of many ecosystems. Parasites can play a role in regulating populations of host species, and they can provide important nutrients to their hosts. Parasites are complex organisms that can have a significant impact on human health and history. Understanding the biology and ecology of parasites is essential for developing effective strategies for controlling parasitic infections and improving human health.

Eliminating parasites is crucial for overall health, as parasites can cause a wide range of health problems. Parasites can interfere with normal body functions, leading to malabsorption of nutrients, anemia, digestive disorders, and even organ failure. They can also weaken the immune system, making individuals more susceptible to other infections and illnesses.

While some parasites may not cause noticeable symptoms, others can cause severe symptoms and even life-threatening conditions. For example, the tapeworm can grow to be several meters long and can cause grave damage to the digestive system, while the liver fluke can cause liver damage and increase the risk of liver cancer.

Besides causing health problems, parasites can also damage the quality of life. Parasitic infections can cause fatigue, depression, and anxiety, and can make it difficult to conduct daily activities.

To prevent and eliminate parasitic infections, it is important to do a parasite cleansing every year. A parasite cleanse involves using natural remedies or anti-parasitic medications to eliminate parasites from the body. This can help improve overall health and reduce the risk of parasitic infections.

Doing a parasite cleanse can also help identify any underlying health problems. If symptoms persist after a parasite cleanse, it may indicate a more serious underlying health issue that requires medical attention.

In addition to doing a parasite cleanse, it is also important to practice good hygiene and maintain a healthy lifestyle to prevent parasitic infections. This includes washing hands regularly, washing fruits and vegetables thoroughly, and avoiding contaminated food and water.

Eliminating parasites is essential for overall health and well-being. Doing a parasite cleanse every year can help eliminate parasitic infections and prevent future infections, leading to improved health and quality of life. It is important to take steps to prevent parasitic infections and seek medical attention if symptoms persist.

CHAPTER 1:
UNDERSTANDING PARASITES

Types of parasites and their effects on the body

Several types of parasites can affect the human body. Some of the most common types of parasites include protozoa, helminths, and ectoparasites. Each type of parasite has its unique characteristics and effects on the body.

Protozoa are single-celled organisms that can cause a wide range of infections in humans. These parasites can be found in contaminated food and water, and they can cause illnesses such as giardiasis, cryptosporidiosis, and toxoplasmosis. Protozoa can infect various parts of the body, including the intestines, liver, and bloodstream.

Helminths are multi-cellular parasites that can range in size from a few millimeters to several meters long. These parasites can be found in contaminated soil or water, and they can infect humans through the skin, mouth, or anus. Common types of helminths include roundworms, tapeworms, and flukes. Helminths can cause a wide range of symptoms, including digestive problems, anemia, malnutrition, and even organ failure.

Ectoparasites are parasites that live on

the outside of the body, such as lice, ticks, and fleas. These parasites can cause a wide range of problems, including skin irritation, itching, and the transmission of infectious diseases such as Lyme disease and typhus.

Parasites can have various effects on the body depending on the type of parasite and the location of infection. Some parasites can cause mild symptoms, such as diarrhea and abdominal pain, while others can cause severe symptoms such as organ failure and even death. In addition to physical symptoms, parasites can also hurt mental health, causing anxiety, depression, and other mood disorders.

Parasitic infections can also increase the risk of other health problems. For example, infections with certain types of parasites have been linked to an increased risk of certain cancers, such as liver cancer and bladder cancer. Parasitic infections can also weaken the immune system, making individuals more susceptible to other infections and illnesses.

Common symptoms of parasite infections

Parasite infections can cause a wide range of symptoms that can vary depending on the type of parasite and the location of the infection. However, some common symptoms of parasite infections have been identified through research.

1. Digestive problems: Parasite infections can cause a range of digestive problems, including diarrhea, constipation, nausea, vomiting, and abdominal pain. These symptoms can be caused by parasites infecting the intestines or other parts of the digestive system.

2. Fatigue: Parasite infections can cause fatigue, weakness, and lethargy. This may be due to the body's immune response to the infection, as well as the parasite's effect on nutrient absorption.

3. Anemia: Parasites that feed on blood, such as hookworms, can cause anemia, a condition in which the body does not have enough red blood cells. Anemia can cause fatigue, weakness, and other symptoms.

4. Skin problems: Parasites such as lice, ticks, and fleas can cause skin irritation, itching, and rashes. Parasitic infections can also cause skin infections and lesions.

5. Respiratory problems: Parasitic infections can cause respiratory symptoms such as coughing, wheezing, and shortness of breath. This may be due to parasites infecting the lungs or airways.

6. Joint and muscle pain: Some parasitic infections can cause joint and muscle pain, as well as inflammation. This can be due to the body's immune response to the infection.

7. Mental health problems: Parasite infections can harm mental health, causing symptoms such as anxiety, depression, and other mood disorders.

It is important to note that not all parasitic infections will cause noticeable symptoms. Some individuals may be asymptomatic carriers of parasites, meaning they have the parasite in their body but do not experience any symptoms. However, if symptoms are present, it is important to seek medical attention for proper diagnosis and treatment.

How parasites enter the body and spread

Parasites can enter the body through various routes and spread to distinct parts of the body. Understanding how parasites enter and spread in the body can help individuals take steps to prevent infection.

1. Ingestion: various parasites enter the body through contaminated food and water. This can happen when fecal matter containing parasite eggs or cysts contaminates food or water sources. Ingestion of undercooked or raw meat or fish can also result in parasite infection.

2. Skin contact: Some parasites can enter the body through the skin. For example, the parasite that causes schistosomiasis enters the body when individuals encounter contaminated water, such as when swimming or bathing.

3. Insect bites: Parasites such as malaria and West Nile virus are spread through the bites of infected mosquitoes. Other insects, such as ticks and fleas, can also transmit parasitic infections.

4. Sexual contact: Parasites can also be spread through sexual contact. For example, trichomoniasis is a sexually transmitted parasitic infection.

Once parasites enter the body, they can spread to distinct parts of the body through the bloodstream or by migrating through tissues. Some parasites, such as tapeworms, can grow to several meters and can spread to distinct parts of the body through the digestive system.

Parasites can also spread from person to person through direct or indirect contact. For example, pinworms, which are commonly found in children, can be spread from person to person through contaminated bedding, clothing, or other items.

In conclusion, parasites can enter the body through various routes and spread to various parts of the body. Taking steps to prevent parasite infection, such as practicing good hygiene, avoiding contaminated food and water sources, and protecting against insect bites, can help reduce the risk of infection. If the parasitic infection is suspected, prompt diagnosis and treatment are essential to prevent the further spread of the infection.

Diagnostic tests for detecting parasites

Several diagnostic tests can detect parasites in the body. These tests can help identify the type of parasite causing the infection and guide treatment decisions.

1. Stool examination: A stool examination is a common test used to detect parasites that infect the intestines. This test involves collecting a stool sample and examining it under a microscope for parasite eggs or cysts.

2. Blood tests: Blood tests can detect parasites that infect the blood, such as malaria and Babesia. These tests can also measure antibody levels to certain parasites, which can help diagnose chronic infections.

3. Imaging tests: Imaging tests such as X-rays, CT scans, and ultrasounds can detect certain types of parasites, such as tapeworms and liver flukes. These tests can also help identify the location and extent of the infection.

4. Biopsy: In some cases, a tissue biopsy may be necessary to diagnose a parasitic infection. This involves taking a small sample of tissue from the affected area and examining it under a microscope for parasites.

5. Serological tests: Serological tests measure the levels of antibodies in the blood against specific parasites. These tests can help diagnose chronic infections and can be useful in monitoring treatment.

It is important to note that diagnostic tests for parasites can sometimes produce false-negative results, especially if the infection is in its initial stages or if the parasite is not present in the area being tested. Repeat testing may be necessary if initial test results are negative but symptoms persist.

There are several diagnostic tests available for detecting parasites. The choice of test will depend on the suspected type and location of the infection. Early diagnosis and treatment of parasitic infections are important for preventing the further spread of the infection and minimizing complications.

CHAPTER 2: NATURAL REMEDIES FOR ELIMINATING PARASITES

Foods that help eliminate parasites

The food that we eat in our daily life will determine our health, here are some specific foods that can control parasitic infections, incorporating certain foods into the diet can help support the body's natural ability to eliminate parasites. Here are some foods that may be helpful:

1. Garlic: Garlic has natural anti-parasitic properties and can help eliminate parasites in the gut. It can be eaten raw, cooked, or taken as a supplement.
2. Pumpkin seeds: Pumpkin seeds are rich in an amino acid called cucurbitacin, which has been shown to have anti-parasitic properties. Eating raw or roasted pumpkin seeds may help eliminate parasites in the intestines.
3. Pineapple: Pineapple contains an enzyme called bromelain, which has been shown to have anti-parasitic properties. Eating fresh pineapple or taking a bromelain supplement may help eliminate parasites.
4. Coconut oil: Coconut oil contains medium-chain fatty acids that have been shown to have anti-parasitic properties. Adding coconut oil to the diet may help eliminate parasites in the gut.
5. Fermented foods: Fermented foods such as kimchi, sauerkraut, and kefir contain beneficial bacteria that can help promote a healthy gut microbiome. A healthy gut microbiome can help support the body's natural ability to eliminate parasites.
6. Papaya: Papaya contains an enzyme called papain, which has been shown to have anti-parasitic properties. Eating

> fresh papaya or taking a papain supplement may help eliminate parasites.

7. Turmeric: Turmeric has natural anti-inflammatory and anti-parasitic properties. Adding turmeric to the diet may help eliminate parasites and reduce inflammation in the body.

It is important to note that while these foods may help support the body's natural ability to eliminate parasites, they should not be used as a substitute for medical treatment. If a parasitic infection is suspected, it is important to seek medical attention for proper diagnosis and treatment.

Herbal remedies for parasite cleansing

Herbal remedies for parasite cleansing have been used for centuries in various cultures around the world. Parasites are organisms that live inside or on a host organism and can cause a range of health problems, including digestive issues, fatigue, and weakened immune function. Herbal remedies have been traditionally used to help eliminate parasites from the body and support overall health

One of the most used herbs for parasite cleansing is wormwood (Artemisia absinthium). Wormwood contains a compound called absinthin, which is effective against a variety of parasites, including giardia and pinworms. Wormwood is often used in combination with other herbs, such as black walnut and cloves, to create a powerful parasite cleanse.

Black walnut (Juglans nigra) is another popular herb for parasite cleansing. The outer hull of the black walnut contains a substance called juglone, which is effective against a variety of parasites, including tapeworms and roundworms. Black walnut is often combined with wormwood and cloves to create a comprehensive parasite cleanse.

Cloves (Syzygium aromaticum) are another powerful herb for parasite cleansing. Cloves contain a compound called eugenol, which is effective against a variety of parasites, including giardia and tapeworms. Cloves are often combined with wormwood and black walnut to create a comprehensive parasite cleanse.

In addition to these three herbs, many other herbs can be used for parasite cleansing, including garlic (Allium sativum), oregano (Origanum vulgare), and thyme (Thymus vulgaris). These herbs contain compounds that are effective against a range of parasites and can be used alone or in combination with other herbs for a comprehensive parasite cleanse.

It is important to note that herbal remedies should not be used as a substitute for medical treatment. If you suspect that you have a parasite infection, it is important to consult with a healthcare provider to determine the most appropriate treatment plan.

Herbal remedies can be a powerful tool for parasite cleansing and supporting overall health. Wormwood, black walnut, and cloves are three of the most effective herbs for parasite cleansing, but many other herbs can be used as well. When using herbal remedies, it is important to do so under the guidance of a healthcare provider to ensure safe and effective use.

Essential oils for killing parasites

Essential oils have been used for centuries for their therapeutic properties. Some essential oils have also been shown to have antimicrobial properties, including the ability to kill parasites One of the most effective essential oils for killing parasites is oregano oil (Origanum vulgare). Oregano oil contains carvacrol and thymol, two compounds that have been demonstrated to have strong antimicrobial properties. In a study published in the Journal of Applied Microbiology, oregano oil was effective against a range of parasites, including giardia and cryptosporidium.

Another essential oil with strong antimicrobial properties is tea tree oil (Melaleuca alternifolia). Tea tree oil contains terpinen-4-ol, a compound that has demonstrated to have antiparasitic properties. In a study published in the Journal of Parasitology Research, tea tree oil was effective against a range of parasites, including trichomonas vaginalis and Leishmania major.

Clove oil (Syzygium aromaticum) is another essential oil with antiparasitic properties. Clove oil contains eugenol, a compound that has demonstrated to have antiparasitic activity. In a study published in the Journal of Parasitology Research, clove oil was effective against giardia and cryptosporidium. Lemongrass oil (Cymbopogon citratus) has also been shown to have antiparasitic properties.

Lemongrass oil contains citral, a compound that has been shown to have antimicrobial activity. In a study published in the Journal of Essential Oil Research, lemongrass oil was effective against giardia.

Besides these essential oils, many others have been shown to have antiparasitic properties, including cinnamon oil (Cinnamomum zeylanicum), peppermint oil (Mentha x piperita), and thyme oil (Thymus vulgaris).

It is important to note that essential oils should not be used as a substitute for medical treatment. If you suspect that you have a parasite infection, it is important to consult with a healthcare provider to determine the most appropriate treatment plan.

Essential oils can be a powerful tool for killing parasites. Oregano oil, tea tree oil, clove oil, and lemongrass oil are just a few examples of essential oils with antiparasitic properties. When using essential oils, it is important to do so under the guidance of a healthcare provider to ensure

safe and effective use.

Natural supplements to support parasite elimination

Parasite infections are a common health concern, particularly in developing countries with poor sanitation practices. They have indicated natural supplements to support parasite elimination and promote overall health. One of the most effective natural supplements for parasite elimination is probiotics. Probiotics are live bacteria and yeasts that are beneficial to the body, particularly for digestive health. Probiotics work by promoting a healthy gut microbiome, which can help to eliminate parasites from the body. In a study published in the Journal of Clinical Gastroenterology, probiotics were effective against giardia, a common parasite.

Another natural supplement that can support parasite elimination is digestive enzymes. Digestive enzymes are proteins that break food into smaller molecules for absorption. They can also help to break down the protective outer layer of parasites, making them easier to eliminate from the body. In a study published in the Journal of Clinical and Diagnostic Research, digestive enzymes were effective against tapeworms.

Herbal supplements can also be effective in supporting parasite elimination. Black walnut (Juglans nigra) is an herbal supplement that has been traditionally used to eliminate parasites from the body. Black walnut contains a substance called juglone, which is effective against a variety of parasites, including tapeworms and roundworms.

Garlic (Allium sativum) is another herbal supplement that can support parasite elimination. Garlic contains a compound called allicin, which has been shown to have antimicrobial properties. In a study published in the Journal of Medicinal Food, garlic was found to be effective against a variety of parasites, including giardia, cryptosporidium, and entamoeba.

In addition to these supplements, many others can support parasite elimination, including grapefruit seed extract, papaya seed extract, and berberine. These supplements contain compounds that have been shown to have antimicrobial properties, which can help to eliminate parasites from the body.

It is important to note that natural supplements should not be used as a substitute for medical treatment. If you suspect that you have a parasite infection, it is important to consult with a healthcare provider to determine the most appropriate treatment plan.

Natural supplements can be a powerful tool for supporting parasite elimination and promoting overall health. Probiotics, digestive enzymes, black walnut, garlic, and other supplements contain compounds that have been shown to have antimicrobial properties and can help to eliminate parasites from the body. When using natural supplements, it is important to do so under the guidance of a healthcare provider to ensure safe and effective use.

Home remedies for
parasite infections

Parasite infections are a common health issue that affects millions of people worldwide. While medical treatment is necessary for severe cases, several home remedies can be effective in managing mild parasite infections.

Garlic is a common household ingredient that has been traditionally used for centuries to treat various health issues, including parasite infections. Garlic contains an active ingredient called allicin that has antimicrobial properties, which help to kill parasites. In a study published in the Journal of Medicinal Food, garlic was found to be effective against several parasites, including giardia, cryptosporidium, and entamoeba. To use garlic as a home remedy, one can eat raw garlic, add it to meals or consume garlic supplements.

Pumpkin seeds are another popular home remedy for treating parasite infections. Pumpkin seeds contain a compound called cucurbitacin that is believed to paralyze the parasites, making it easier for the body to eliminate them. A study published in the Journal of Medicinal Food found that pumpkin seeds were effective against tapeworms. To use pumpkin seeds as a home remedy, one can consume them raw, roasted, or make pumpkin seed tea.

Papaya is a tropical fruit that has been found to have anthelmintic properties, meaning it helps to eliminate parasitic worms from the body. Papaya contains an enzyme called papain that helps to digest protein, which is the primary source of food for parasitic worms. In a study published in the Journal of Medicinal Plants, papaya was found to be effective against tapeworms. To use papaya as a home remedy, one can consume it raw, blend it into a smoothie, or consume papaya seed extract.

Turmeric is a spice that has anti-inflammatory and antimicrobial properties, which make it an effective home remedy for parasite infections. In a study published in the Journal of Parasitic Diseases, turmeric was found to be effective against giardia. To use turmeric as a home remedy, one can add it to meals, take turmeric supplements, or consume it as tea.

Cloves are another commonly used home remedy for parasite infections. Cloves contain a compound called eugenol that has antiparasitic properties. In a study published in the Journal of Ethnopharmacology, cloves were found to be effective against several types of parasites, including giardia and cryptosporidium. To use cloves as a home remedy, one can consume them as a spice, add them to tea or consume clove oil supplements.

Home remedies can be an effective way to manage mild parasite infections. Garlic, pumpkin seeds, papaya, turmeric, and cloves are just a few examples of home remedies that are effective against a variety of parasites. While home remedies can be helpful, it is important to consult with a healthcare provider if you suspect that you have a parasite infection, as some infections may require medical treatment.

CHAPTER 3: MEDICAL TREATMENTS FOR PARASITE INFECTIONS

Prescription medications for parasite infections

Parasite infections can be severe, and in some cases, require prescription medications to effectively manage and eliminate the infection.

1. Metronidazole: Metronidazole is an antibiotic that is commonly used to treat bacterial infections, but it is also effective against several types of parasites, including giardia and trichomoniasis. Metronidazole works by damaging the DNA of the parasite, preventing it from reproducing and ultimately leading to its death. Some common side effects of metronidazole include nausea, vomiting, and diarrhea.

2. Albendazole: Albendazole is an anthelmintic medication that is commonly used to treat parasitic infections, such as tapeworms, roundworms, and hookworms. Albendazole works by disrupting the parasite's metabolism, causing it to starve and ultimately leading to its death. Some common side effects of albendazole include headache, abdominal pain, and nausea.

3. Ivermectin: Ivermectin is another anthelmintic medication that is commonly used to treat parasitic infections, such as river blindness and scabies. Ivermectin works by paralyzing the parasite's nervous system, making it easier for the body to eliminate it. Some common side effects of ivermectin include dizziness, headache, and diarrhea.

4. Praziquantel: Praziquantel is an anthelmintic medication that is commonly used to treat parasitic infections, such as tapeworms and flukes. Praziquantel works by causing the muscles of the parasite to contract, which leads to its expulsion from the body. Some

common side effects of praziquantel include headache, nausea, and dizziness.

5. Nitazoxanide: Nitazoxanide is an antiparasitic medication that is commonly used to treat infections caused by cryptosporidium and giardia. Nitazoxanide works by disrupting the metabolism of the parasite, causing it to starve and ultimately leading to its death. Some common side effects of nitazoxanide include headache, abdominal pain, and nausea.

In conclusion, prescription medications can be an effective way to manage and eliminate parasitic infections. Metronidazole, albendazole, ivermectin, praziquantel, and nitazoxanide are just a few examples of prescription medications that are commonly used to treat parasite infections. While these medications can be effective, it is important to consult with a healthcare provider before taking any prescription medication, as they may have potential side effects and interactions with other medications.

Side effects of prescription medications

Prescription medications are designed to help manage and treat various medical conditions. However, like any medication, prescription drugs can also come with potential side effects. Gastrointestinal Side Effects: Many prescription medications can cause gastrointestinal side effects such as nausea, vomiting, diarrhea, and constipation. For example, metronidazole, a medication commonly used to treat bacterial and parasitic infections, is known to cause nausea, vomiting, and diarrhea.

1. Cardiovascular Side Effects: Some prescription medications can also cause cardiovascular side effects such as high blood pressure, low blood pressure, and arrhythmia. For example, amphetamines, a type of medication used to treat attention deficit hyperactivity disorder (ADHD), can increase heart rate and blood pressure.

2. Central Nervous System Side Effects: Prescription medications can also affect the central nervous system, leading to side effects such as dizziness, headaches, and seizures. For example, opioids, a type of medication used to manage pain, can cause dizziness, sedation, and respiratory depression.

3. Dermatological Side Effects: Some prescription medications can cause dermatological side effects such as rash, hives, and photosensitivity. For example, tetracycline antibiotics used to treat bacterial infections

can cause photosensitivity and skin rashes.

4. Hepatic and Renal Side Effects: Prescription medications can also affect the liver and kidneys, leading to side effects such as liver damage and kidney failure. For example, statins used to manage high cholesterol can cause liver damage in some individuals.

5. Psychological Side Effects: Some prescription medications can also have psychological side effects such as depression, anxiety, and hallucinations. For example, corticosteroids used to treat inflammation and autoimmune diseases can cause mood changes and depression.

In conclusion, prescription medications can cause a wide range of potential side effects. It is important to consult with a healthcare provider before taking any prescription medication and to monitor for any side effects that may occur. While side effects can concern, various medications are still safe and effective when taken as prescribed. If you experience any concerning side effects, be sure to discuss them with your healthcare provider.

Alternative medical treatments for parasite infections

Alternative medical treatments for parasite infections refer to non-conventional methods of managing and treating parasitic infections. They can use these treatments alongside or instead of conventional prescription medication.

Herbal Remedies: Herbal remedies have been used for centuries to manage and treat various medical conditions, including parasitic infections. Examples of herbs that are commonly used for parasite infections include wormwood, black walnut, and clove. These herbs contain natural compounds that have anti-parasitic properties and can help to eliminate parasites from the body.

1. Essential Oils: Essential oils are concentrated plant extracts that contain potent anti-parasitic compounds. Some of the most effective essential oils for parasite infections include oregano, thyme, and tea tree oil. These oils can be used topically or ingested to help eliminate parasites from the body.

2. Probiotics: Probiotics are beneficial bacteria that live in the gut and help to maintain a healthy balance of microorganisms. Research has indicated that certain strains of probiotics, such as lactobacillus and bifidobacterium, can help to eliminate parasitic infections by boosting the immune system and restoring gut health.

3. Acupuncture: Acupuncture is an ancient Chinese medical practice that involves inserting thin needles into specific points on the body. This practice has been shown to help improve immune function and reduce inflammation, which can help to eliminate parasitic infections.

4. Hydrotherapy: Hydrotherapy involves the use of water for therapeutic purposes. This can include drinking water that has been treated with anti-parasitic herbs or soaking in a bath with essential oils that have anti-parasitic properties.

It is important to note that alternative medical treatments should not be used as a substitute for conventional prescription medication. However, they can be used as complementary therapy to help manage and treat parasitic infections. Before using any alternative medical treatment, it is important to consult with a healthcare provider to ensure that it is safe and appropriate for your individual needs. It is important to note that alternative medical treatments have not been extensively studied, and their effectiveness may vary from person to person.

Safety precautions when taking prescription medications

Prescription medications are a vital component of modern medicine, helping millions of people worldwide manage and treat various medical conditions. However, it is important to understand that prescription medications can also be potentially harmful if not taken with appropriate safety precautions.

Firstly, it is important to understand that prescription medications should only be taken as prescribed by a healthcare provider. This means taking the medication at the recommended dosage, frequency, and duration. Overdosing or underdosing can result in serious health consequences, including organ damage, overdose, and death.

Secondly, it is important to be aware of potential side effects and drug interactions when taking prescription medications. Many medications can interact with other medications, supplements, and foods, leading to potentially harmful side effects. It is important to inform your healthcare provider of all medications, supplements, and foods that you are currently taking to avoid any potential interactions.

Thirdly, it is important to never share prescription medications with others. Prescription medications are prescribed based on individual medical needs, and what is safe and effective for one person may not be safe for another. Sharing prescription medications can lead to serious health consequences and is illegal.

Fourthly, it is important to store prescription medications properly. Many medications can become less effective or even harmful if stored improperly. For example, medications should be kept in a cool, dry place, away from sunlight and moisture. Additionally, medications should be stored out of reach of children and pets to prevent accidental ingestion. Finally, it is important to dispose of prescription medications properly. Many medications can be harmful if disposed of improperly, leading to environmental contamination and potential harm to wildlife. It is important to follow proper disposal guidelines, such as returning unused medications to a pharmacy or participating in a drug take-back program.

Safety precautions when taking prescription medications are crucial to prevent potential harm and ensure safe and effective treatment. By following these safety precautions, we can ensure that prescription medications are used safely and effectively to manage and treat medical conditions. It is important to consult with a healthcare provider if you have any concerns or questions regarding prescription medications.

CHAPTER 4: DETOXIFICATION AND CLEANSING

The importance of detoxifying the body

Detoxification refers to the process of eliminating harmful toxins from the body. While our body has natural detoxification processes, exposure to environmental toxins, unhealthy diets, and other factors can compromise these processes. This is why it is important to detoxify the body at least once a year.

Firstly, detoxifying the body can help improve overall health and well-being. Accumulation of toxins in the body can lead to a range of health problems, including fatigue, headaches, digestive issues, and skin problems. By eliminating toxins from the body, we can help improve our overall health and reduce the risk of developing these health problems.

Secondly, detoxifying the body can help boost the immune system. Toxins in the body can compromise immune function, making us more susceptible to infections and other illnesses. By eliminating toxins from the body, we can help improve immune function, leading to better overall health and a reduced risk of developing infections and other illnesses.

Thirdly, detoxifying the body can help

improve digestion and nutrient absorption. Toxins in the body can disrupt digestive processes, leading to digestive issues such as bloating, constipation, and diarrhea. By eliminating toxins from the body, we can help improve digestive function and nutrient absorption, leading to better overall health.

Fourthly, detoxifying the body can help improve mental health. Toxins in the body can affect brain function, leading to cognitive issues such as brain fog and memory problems. By eliminating toxins from the body, we can help improve brain function and reduce the risk of developing cognitive issues.

Finally, detoxifying the body can help improve skin health. Toxins in the body can affect skin health, leading to issues such as acne, eczema, and psoriasis. By eliminating toxins from the body, we can help improve skin health, leading to clearer, healthier skin.

Detoxifying the body at least once a year is crucial for maintaining overall health and well-being. By eliminating harmful toxins from the body, we can improve immune function, digestion, nutrient absorption, mental health, and skin health. It is important to consult with a healthcare provider to determine the best detoxification method for your individual needs.

Methods for detoxification and cleansing

Detoxification and cleansing refer to the process of removing harmful toxins from the body. While our body has natural detoxification processes, exposure to environmental toxins, unhealthy diets, and other factors can compromise these processes. There are several methods for detoxification and cleansing, each with its benefits and drawbacks.

The first method for detoxification and cleansing is a juice cleanse. Juice cleanses involve drinking only fresh vegetable and fruit juices for a set period, usually 3-10 days. This method is popular because it is easy to follow and can help flush out toxins from the body. Juices are also rich in vitamins, minerals, and antioxidants, which can help improve overall health.

The second method for detoxification and cleansing is water fast. Water fasts involve consuming only water for a set period, usually 1-3 days. This method is more challenging than juice cleanses, but it can be more effective at eliminating toxins from the body. Water fasts also allow the digestive system to rest, which can improve overall health.

The third method for detoxification and cleansing is a colon cleanse. Colon cleanses involve flushing out the colon with water or other fluids. This method can help remove toxins from the colon and improve digestive function. However, it can also be harsh on the body and may cause discomfort.

The fourth method for detoxification and cleansing is a sauna. Saunas involve sitting in a heated room for a set period, usually 10-20 minutes. This method can help eliminate toxins through sweating and improve circulation. Saunas are also relaxing and can help reduce stress.

The fifth method for detoxification and cleansing is a liver cleanse. Liver cleanses involve consuming specific foods and supplements to support liver function and eliminate toxins from the body. This method can help improve liver function and overall health, but it should only be done under the guidance of a healthcare provider. In conclusion, there are several methods for detoxification and cleansing, each with its benefits and drawbacks. Juice cleanses, water fasts, colon cleanses, saunas and liver cleanses are all effective methods for eliminating toxins from the body and improving overall health. It is important to consult with a healthcare provider before starting any detoxification or cleansing program to determine the best method for your individual needs.

Benefits of detoxification for parasite elimination

Detoxification is the process of removing harmful toxins from the body, and it is an essential component of overall health and wellness. When it comes to parasitic infections, detoxification is even more critical as it helps the body eliminate the parasites and the toxins that they produce.

First, detoxification can help to eliminate parasites and their eggs from the body. When the body is overloaded with toxins, it becomes a breeding ground for parasites. By eliminating these toxins, detoxification can create an environment that is hostile to parasites, preventing them from thriving in the body. This can help to reduce the risk of infection, as well as reduce the severity of existing infections.

Detoxification can also help to boost the immune system, which is essential for fighting off parasitic infections. When the body is overloaded with toxins, the immune system becomes weakened, making it easier for parasites to invade and take hold. By removing these toxins, detoxification can help to strengthen the immune system, making it more effective at identifying and eliminating parasites from the body.

Another benefit of detoxification is improved digestive function. Parasitic infections can wreak havoc on the digestive system, causing a range of symptoms, including diarrhea, constipation, and bloating. Detoxification can help to restore balance to the digestive system, promoting regularity and reducing symptoms of discomfort.

Detoxification can also help to improve overall health and wellness. When the body is free from toxins, it can function at its best, with more energy, better sleep, and improved mental clarity. This can have a positive impact on all aspects of life, from work to personal relationships.

Detoxification is a powerful tool for eliminating parasites from the body and improving overall health and wellness. By removing toxins, detoxification can create an environment that is hostile to parasites, boost the immune system, improve digestive function, and promote overall health. If you are struggling with a parasitic infection, consider incorporating detoxification into your treatment plan for the best possible outcome.

CHAPTER 5: RESTORING HEALTH AFTER PARASITE INFECTIONS

Nutritional strategies
for restoring health

Nutrition is a critical component of overall health and wellness, and it plays a vital role in restoring health after an illness or injury. Primarily, it is essential to focus on a balanced and varied diet that includes plenty of fruits, vegetables, whole grains, lean protein, and healthy fats. These foods provide the body with the essential nutrients it needs to heal and recover, including vitamins, minerals, antioxidants, and fiber.

One specific nutrient that is crucial for restoring health is protein. Protein is essential for repairing damaged tissues and building new cells. Useful sources of protein include lean meats, fish, eggs, beans, nuts, and seeds.

Another important nutrient for restoring health is omega-3 fatty acids. These healthy fats are anti-inflammatory and can help to reduce inflammation in the body, which is essential for healing. Useful sources of omega-3s include fatty fish, flaxseeds, chia seeds, and walnuts.

Besides focusing on specific nutrients, it is also essential to focus on overall calorie intake. When the body is healing, it requires more energy to support the healing process. It is important to consume enough calories to provide the body with the energy it needs to repair and recover.

Finally, it is essential to avoid processed foods and foods high in sugar and saturated fat. These foods can increase inflammation in the body, which can interfere with the healing process. Instead, focus on whole, nutrient-dense foods that support health and wellness.

In conclusion, nutrition is a critical component of restoring health after an illness or injury. By focusing on a balanced and varied diet that includes plenty of fruits, vegetables, whole grains, lean protein, and healthy fats, as well as specific nutrients like protein and omega-3s, we can support the healing process and promote overall health and wellness. If you are looking to restore your health, consider incorporating these nutritional strategies into your lifestyle for the best possible outcome.

Exercise and physical activity for restoring health

Exercise and physical activity are essential components of overall health and wellness, and they play a vital role in restoring health after an illness or injury.

First, exercise and physical activity can help to improve cardiovascular health, which is essential for restoring health after an illness or injury. Regular exercise can help to strengthen the heart and improve circulation, which can help to deliver oxygen and nutrients to the body's tissues more efficiently. This can support the healing process and promote overall health and wellness.

Another benefit of exercise and physical activity is improved muscle strength and flexibility. When the body is healing, it is essential to maintain or improve muscle strength and flexibility to support mobility and prevent further injury. Activities such as weightlifting, yoga, and Pilates can be particularly beneficial for improving strength and flexibility.

Exercise and physical activity can also help to reduce stress and anxiety, which is essential for restoring health. Stress and anxiety can interfere with the healing process, and they can also exacerbate existing health conditions. Exercise and physical activity can help to reduce stress and anxiety, promoting relaxation and improving overall mental health and well-being.

In addition to these benefits, exercise and physical activity can also improve overall energy levels, improve sleep quality, and support weight management, all of which can contribute to overall health and wellness.

Examples of activities that can support the healing process include walking, cycling, swimming, dancing, and tai chi. These activities are minimal impact, making them ideal for individuals who are recovering from an illness or injury. They can also be tailored to meet the individual's needs, allowing for a customized approach to exercise and physical activity.

Exercise and physical activity are essential components of restoring health after an illness or injury. Improving cardiovascular health, muscle strength, and flexibility, reducing stress and anxiety, improving energy levels and sleep quality, and supporting weight management, exercise, and physical activity can promote overall health and wellness. If you are looking to restore your health, consider incorporating exercise and physical activity into your daily routine for the best possible outcome.

Mind-body techniques for promoting healing

The mind and body are interconnected, and this relationship can play a significant role in promoting healing. Mind-body techniques are practices that can help to harness the power of the mind to support physical healing.

Primarily, mind-body techniques can help to reduce stress and anxiety, which is essential for promoting healing. Stress and anxiety can interfere with the healing process, and they can also exacerbate existing health conditions. Mind-body techniques such as meditation, deep breathing, and mindfulness can help to reduce stress and anxiety, promoting relaxation and improving overall mental health and well-being.

Another benefit of mind-body techniques is improved pain management. Pain can be a significant barrier to healing and managing pain effectively can help to support the healing process. Mind-body techniques such as hypnosis, guided imagery, and acupuncture can be effective in managing pain and supporting the healing process.

Mind-body techniques can also help to improve sleep quality, which is essential for promoting healing. Sleep is a critical component of the healing process and getting enough restful sleep can help to support physical and mental health. Mind-body techniques such as yoga, progressive muscle relaxation, and biofeedback can be effective in improving sleep quality.

In addition to these benefits, mind-body techniques can also improve overall mood and emotional well-being, support healthy habits, and improve the overall quality of life. Examples of mind-body techniques that can support healing include meditation, yoga, acupuncture, hypnosis, biofeedback, guided imagery, deep breathing, and progressive muscle relaxation. These practices are evidence-based and can be tailored to meet the individual's needs, allowing for a customized approach to healing.

In conclusion, mind-body techniques are powerful tools for promoting healing. By reducing stress and anxiety, improving pain management, improving sleep quality, improving mood and emotional well-being, supporting healthy habits, and improving the overall quality of life, mind-body techniques can support the healing process in multiple ways. If you are looking to support your healing process, consider incorporating mind-body techniques into your daily routine for the best possible

outcome.

Medical treatments for addressing long-term effects of parasite infections

Parasite infections can have long-term effects on the body, even after the parasites themselves have been eliminated. These long-term effects can include chronic inflammation, autoimmune disorders, and nutrient deficiencies. Fortunately, there are medical treatments available to address these long-term effects and support the body's healing process.

One common long-term effect of parasite infections is chronic inflammation. Chronic inflammation can lead to a range of health problems, including joint pain, fatigue, and digestive issues. Medical treatments such as anti-inflammatory medications can help to reduce inflammation and alleviate these symptoms. Additionally, supplements such as omega-3 fatty acids and curcumin can be effective in reducing inflammation and promoting healing.

Autoimmune disorders are another potential long-term effect of parasite infections. Parasites can disrupt the immune system, leading to an overactive immune response that can attack healthy tissues in the body. Medical treatments such as immunosuppressants can help to calm down the immune system and reduce the risk of autoimmune disorders. Additionally, supplements such as vitamin D and probiotics can support immune system function and promote overall health.

Nutrient deficiencies are also a common long-term effect of parasite infections. Parasites can interfere with nutrient absorption, leading to deficiencies in essential vitamins and minerals. Medical treatments such as nutrient supplementation can help to address these deficiencies and support overall health. Additionally, dietary changes and lifestyle modifications can help to promote nutrient absorption and support the body's healing process.

Medical treatments can be highly effective in addressing the long-term effects of parasite infections. By reducing inflammation, addressing autoimmune disorders, and addressing nutrient deficiencies, medical treatments can support the body's healing process and improve overall health and well-being. If you are experiencing the long-term effects of a parasite infection, it is important to seek medical treatment to address these issues and support your body's healing process.

CHAPTER 6: PREVENTION AND MAINTENANCE

Strategies for preventing parasite infections

Parasite infections can be uncomfortable and even dangerous, leading to a range of symptoms and potential long-term health effects. Fortunately, there are strategies that you can use to help prevent parasite infections and protect your health.

One of the most important strategies for preventing parasite infections is to practice good hygiene. This means washing your hands regularly, particularly after using the bathroom or encountering potentially contaminated surfaces. It also means avoiding sharing personal items such as towels or toothbrushes, which can help to prevent the spread of infection. Additionally, it is important to practice safe food handling, including washing fruits and vegetables thoroughly and cooking meat to the appropriate temperature.

Another key strategy for preventing parasite infections is to avoid exposure to potentially contaminated water. This can include drinking bottled water when traveling to areas with questionable water quality and avoiding swimming in bodies of water that may be contaminated. Additionally, it is important to take precautions when traveling to areas with high rates of parasitic infection, including taking medication to prevent infection and using insect repellent to avoid exposure to mosquitoes and other disease-carrying insects.

Supplements and natural remedies can also be effective in preventing parasite infections. Garlic, for example, has been shown to have anti-parasitic properties and can be effective in preventing infection. Additionally, supplements such as probiotics can help to support gut health and boost immune system function, which can help to prevent infection.

There are many strategies that you can use to help prevent parasite infections and protect your health. By practicing good hygiene, avoiding exposure to contaminated water, and taking supplements and natural remedies, you can significantly reduce your risk of infection. If you are traveling to areas with high rates of parasitic infection, it is especially important to take precautions to protect yourself. By taking these steps, you can help to prevent parasite infections and maintain optimal health and well-being.

Foods and supplements that support parasite prevention

Parasite infections can cause a range of unpleasant symptoms and long-term health effects. Fortunately, some foods and supplements can help to support parasite prevention and protect your health.

One of the most effective foods for supporting parasite prevention is garlic. Garlic has been shown to have anti-parasitic properties and can help to prevent infections by inhibiting the growth and reproduction of parasites. Other foods that are high in anti-inflammatory compounds and antioxidants, such as ginger, turmeric, and green tea, can help to boost immune system function and support overall health.

Supplements such as probiotics and digestive enzymes can also be effective in supporting parasite prevention. Probiotics are beneficial bacteria that can help to support gut health, which is important for preventing parasitic infections. Digestive enzymes can help to collapse proteins and other compounds that parasites need to survive, making it more difficult for them to thrive in the body.

Besides specific foods and supplements, it is important to maintain a healthy, balanced diet to support overall health and immune system function. This means consuming a variety of nutrient-dense foods, such as fruits, vegetables, whole grains, and lean proteins. These foods are rich in vitamins, minerals, and other nutrients that are important for maintaining optimal health and preventing infections.

In conclusion, sufficient foods and supplements can help to support parasite prevention and protect your health. By incorporating foods such as garlic, ginger, and green tea into your diet, and taking supplements such as probiotics and digestive enzymes, you can significantly reduce your risk of infection. Maintaining a healthy, balanced diet is important for overall health and immune system function, which can help to prevent a range of health problems, including parasite infections. By taking these steps, you can help to support your health and well-being and prevent parasitic infections.

Practices for maintaining overall health and wellness

Maintaining overall health and wellness is essential for leading a happy and fulfilling life. Many practices can help to support physical, mental, and emotional well-being. In well-being, we will explore the benefits of these practices and provide multiple examples of how to incorporate them into your daily life.

One of the most important practices for maintaining overall health and wellness is regular exercise. They have shown exercise to improve cardiovascular health, reduce stress and anxiety, and promote healthy weight management. Many diverse types of exercise can be effective, including cardio, strength training, and yoga. Incorporating regular exercise into your routine can help you feel more energized and improve your overall sense of well-being.

Another important practice for maintaining overall health and wellness is getting enough rest and sleep. Sleep is essential for physical and mental health, and lack of sleep can contribute to a range of health problems, including obesity, heart disease, and depression. Aim to get at least 7-8 hours of sleep each night and establish a regular sleep schedule to help regulate your body's natural sleep-wake cycle.

In addition to exercise and sleep, it is important to maintain a healthy diet to support overall health and wellness. This means consuming a variety of nutrient-dense foods such as fruits, vegetables, whole grains, and lean proteins. These foods are rich in vitamins, minerals, and other nutrients that are important for maintaining optimal health.

Mental and emotional health is also a critical component of overall health and wellness. Practices such as meditation, mindfulness, and therapy can be effective in promoting mental and emotional well-being. These practices can help to reduce stress and anxiety, improve self-awareness, and promote a sense of calm and balance.

Many practices can help to support overall health and wellness. Regular exercise, getting enough rest and sleep, maintaining a healthy diet, and promoting mental and emotional health through practices such as meditation and therapy are all important strategies. By incorporating these practices into your daily life, you can improve your physical, mental, and emotional well-being and well-being pier, healthier life.

CONCLUSION

Throughout the discussion, we have explored various aspects of parasite infections, including their causes, symptoms, and treatments. We have seen that while prescription medications are effective in treating parasite infections, they often come with side effects that can be harmful to the body. Therefore, natural supplements and home remedies can be used as alternative medical treatments.

In addition, we have explored the importance of detoxification and cleansing for promoting healing and eliminating parasites from the body. Adopting nutritional strategies, exercise routines, and mind-body techniques can also be beneficial in supporting overall health and wellness.

Prevention is the key to avoiding parasite infections. Eating a healthy and balanced diet that includes foods and supplements known to support parasite prevention can reduce the risk of infection. Good hygiene practices, such as washing hands regularly and avoiding contaminated water sources, can also help to prevent parasite infections.

In conclusion, a multifaceted approach that combines medical treatments, preventative measures, and lifestyle practices is necessary to effectively address and prevent parasite infections. By prioritizing one's health and well-being, individuals can lead a fulfilling and healthy life, free from the negative effects of parasitic infections. It is important to stay informed and take the necessary steps to maintain good health and prevent infections from occurring.

Encouragement to act and prioritize health

Taking care of your health is one of the most important things you can do for yourself. It is easy to get caught up in the hustle and bustle of daily life but neglecting your health can lead to grave consequences down the road. Do not wait until you are faced with a health crisis to start prioritizing your well-being.

Commit today to acting and prioritizing your health. This can include simple changes such as incorporating more whole foods into your diet, drinking plenty of water, and engaging in regular exercise. You can also explore different mind-body techniques, such as yoga or meditation, to help manage stress and promote relaxation.

Additionally, it is important to stay informed about potential health risks and take the necessary preventative measures. This can include practicing good hygiene, avoiding high-risk activities, and incorporating foods and supplements known to support immune health and prevent parasitic infections.

Do not let the fear of the unknown or the discomfort of change hold you back from acting. Prioritizing your health is a decision that will pay off overall, both for you and those around you. Take the first step today towards a healthier and happier future.

FINAL THOUGHTS

In today's world, parasites have become a common health concern that affects millions of people worldwide. It is therefore essential to prioritize parasite elimination as a means of promoting optimal health and wellness.

Parasite infections can cause a range of symptoms, including fatigue, digestive issues, and even chronic diseases. By taking steps to eliminate parasites from the body, individuals can experience significant improvements in their overall health and well-being. This can include increased energy levels, better digestion, and a stronger immune system.

There are various strategies and treatments available for parasite elimination, including natural supplements, home remedies, prescription medications, and detoxification methods. It is important to explore and choose the most effective approach for your specific needs and situation.

By incorporating preventative measures and healthy lifestyle practices, individuals can reduce their risk of contracting parasitic infections in the first place. This can include practicing good hygiene, avoiding high-risk activities, and eating a balanced diet that includes foods and supplements known to support immune health.

In conclusion, parasite elimination is an essential component of optimal health and well-being. By acting and prioritizing parasite elimination, individuals can experience significant improvements in their physical and mental health. Do not wait until it is too late - take steps today to eliminate parasites from your body and live a healthy and fulfilling life.

ACKNOWLEDGMENT

I would like to express my deep gratitude and appreciation to all those who have contributed to the creation and success of this project.

First, I would like to thank the individuals who generously shared their knowledge, expertise, and firsthand experiences with me. Your insights and perspectives have been invaluable in shaping the content and direction of this work.

I also extend my appreciation to my family and friends for their unwavering support and encouragement throughout this process. Your belief in me and the importance of this project has been a constant source of motivation and inspiration.

I would like to acknowledge everyone on the team who worked diligently behind the scenes to bring this project to fruition. Your expertise and dedication have helped to create a final product that I am proud to share with the world.

Finally, I would like to express my gratitude to the readers of this book. Your interest and engagement with the content truly make this work meaningful. I hope that the information and insights presented here will help you on your journey toward better health and well-being.

Thank you to all who have played a role in this project. Your contributions have not gone unnoticed and are deeply appreciated.